Intermittent Fasting + Keto Diet

Ketogenic Meal Plans For Intermittent Fasting, The Ultimate Fat Burning Combination

James Brook

Table of Contents

Introduction

Well done and congratulations for downloading your personal copy of,

"Intermittent Fasting + Keto Diet: Ketogenic Meal Plans For Intermittent Fasting, The Ultimate Fat Burning Combination."

Maybe by now you've already heard about the Ketogenic diet and Intermittent fasting, but did you know that you can combine these two? Maybe you do, but you don't know how to do it right. Or maybe you're interested in intermittent fasting but you need a healthy meal plan to follow for the feeding windows. If this sounds like you then this book is perfect for you!

This book will primarily focus on structured ketogenic meal plans, specifying what to eat and when to eat it. We will discuss the feeding window times of the different IF styles and how to fit the ketogenic meal plans into these time slots throughout the week.

Now there's a lot of information out there about all kinds of quick weight-loss tricks, and fad diets. They all tend to make the same promises, claiming that you can achieve perfect health, stunning looks, and a slimmer figure for the rest of your life. The reality is that these are all just short term fixes. If you're committed enough you may be able to achieve the good looks and figure for a little while, but it won't last in the long term. With those types of fad diets you'll never get a true healthy body from them, even if you do lose some of the weight.

People will spend years of their lives trying different diets, and they hardly get any results. In 2007, there was a study performed where they learned that women spend 31 years, on average trying diets, just barely surpassing the men at 28 years.

The next big problem is that diets will typically require major changes in your eating. Many require that you drop your calorie intake drastically. There are some that will require you to eat unappealing and tasteless foods, which will only make you end your diet even faster. This causes them to revert back to the old eating habits.

The diet this book will introduce you to is the ketogenic diet. I assure you this is not one of these 'fad diets', its health benefits are truly tremendous and its principles have been used for decades. In fact, a keto diet is not only a great weight loss strategy, it can also be used for the treatment of different health conditions and can help your body to avoid other types of serious illnesses. There is a reason why the ketogenic diet has gained so much popularity in such a short time.

The journey of this book is separated into intermittent fasting and the ketogenic diet. You will learn the basic information of each, and then we will look at the huge benefits the two of them combined can give you. Afterwards we will move on to the different schedules for your intermittent fasting plan. There will be five different versions, allowing you to decide which one works best for you. And here's where the best part comes in. You will find ketogenic meal plans for each of the intermittent fasting plans and all the breakfast, lunch, and dinner recipes to follow.

Every effort was made to ensure that this book is filled with as much useful information as possible. Please enjoy!

What is Intermittent Fasting?

Intermittent fasting is a popular fitness and health trend throughout the world that dates all the way back to ancient times. People still use it today to lose weight, simplify their lifestyle, and improve their health. Studies have shown that it has great effects on your brain and body. It can even help you to live longer.

Intermittent fasting is not a diet; it's a way to eat. It provides you a schedule of when you have your meals so that you receive the most from them. It doesn't affect the foods that you eat, but just the times that you eat them. Common methods use daily 16-hour fasts or fasting for a complete day two times each week.

This type of fasting proves to be easier to follow than a diet. Diets don't fail because you eat the wrong foods; it's because people tend not to stick to them for a long time. It's not nutritional; it's behavioral. Intermittent fasting is easy once you realize that you don't have to eat all the time and pay so much attention to food. It is a routine that anyone can easily adapt to.

Humans have fasted all throughout evolution. In fact it is a part of religions such as Buddhism, Christianity, and Islam. We may have done this in the past due to the lack of food that was available. Our ancestors didn't have access to refrigerators, stores, or food they could get all year. There were many times where we didn't have anything to eat and our bodies figured out a way to work properly without any source of food for a short period of time.

Fasting is actually more natural than eating three or four meals every day. It is a good way to help you get lean without cutting calories or trying to diet. Your calories will actually stay the same when you fast. Many will eat larger meals within a much shorter time frame. Intermittent fasting keeps muscle mass while helping you get lean.

It is a simple way to take off excess weight while holding onto your good weight, since little to no behavior change is involved. This is great since intermittent fasting is simple enough that you can actually do it and useful enough to still make a powerful difference.

To figure out how this will lead to losing fat, we have to know the difference between the fed and fasted states of the body.

The fed state is when your body is breaking down and absorbing food. This begins when you start to eat food and lasts for about five hours as your body absorbs and digests it. When in this state, it is hard to burn off fat because your insulin levels will be higher.

Eventually, the body enters a post-absorptive state which just means that your body isn't processing foods. This state will last about 12 hours after you eat. This is when the body enters into the fasted state. You can burn fat easier in this state because your insulin is low. Within this state, your body burns fat that hasn't been available to it while in the fed state.

Since it takes around 12 hours to reach the fast state from the last time you ate, it's very rare that they body ever enters this state. This is one reason why people begin to intermittent fast, so we lose fat without having to change what we eat, the amount we eat, or whether or not we exercise. Fasting will put your body into a state of burning fat that you won't enter when eating normally.

Here are the five popular IF methods that we will be discussing in this book:

- **The 5:2 Diet**: Pick two days out of the week that aren't right after the other. Eat just 500 to 600 calories on these days. Eat normally on the other five days.

- **Eat-Stop-Eat**: This means you will fast for 24 hours a couple of times a week. You eat at 6:00 pm one day and won't eat again until 6:00 pm the next day.

- **Alternate-day fasting**: This one works similar to the 5:2 except you alternate low-calorie and normal calorie every day. On your low-cal/fast days, you will eat a fifth of your typical calorie intake. So 400-500 calories.

- **The 16/8 Diet**: This method skips breakfast and restricts your eating time to eight hours. You will eat from 12:00 pm to 8:00 pm. You then stay in a fasted state in the 16 hours between 8:00 pm and 12:00 pm the next day.

- **Lean gains**: For a woman, you fast for 14 hours, and for a man, you fast for 16 hours. This fast happens every night after dinner until afternoon the next day, just like the 16/8 Diet. You'll eat during the remaining eight to ten hours. You are also required to exercise and eat certain things on this plan.

Since all of these methods involve consistent fasting, or eating fewer calories, you should be able to lose weight on any of them, as long as you don't eat too much unhealthy food during your eating times.

Most people tend to find that the 16/8 method is the easiest one to stick with, but the one that will suit your lifestyle the best is totally up to you. We will be discussing these five intermittent fasting plans in further detail later on in the book.

When fasting, several things happen to your body on the molecular and cellular levels. Your body will change your hormone levels in order to allow itself to have access to your stored fat. The cells will repair themselves through the process of 'autophagy' and change your genes.

Here are some healthy changes that can happen when you fast:

- **Gene expression**: You will experience changes in the way that your genes function relating to protecting you against disease and longevity.

- **Cellular repair**: When in the fasting state, your cells will start repairing. This is called 'autophagy', in which the cells remove dysfunctional and old proteins that get built up in your cells.

- **Insulin**: Level of insulin drop excessively and insulin sensitivity improves. Lower levels of insulin will make body fat more accessible.

- **Human Growth Hormone**: Human growth hormone levels will greatly increase. This benefits muscle gain and fat loss.

These changes in gene expression, cellular function, and hormone levels, attribute to a multitude of health benefits.

The most obvious one being, losing a lot of fat. This natural weight loss is the main reason why people use intermittent fasting. Since you eat fewer meals, fasting significantly reduces the number of calories that are consumed. The body will also change your hormone levels while fasting in order to further help with losing more weight.

Besides lowering insulin levels and raising the amount of growth hormones, it will also create an increase in norepinephrine, which is a fat burning hormone. Because of these hormone changes, fasting might increase your metabolic rate by anywhere from 3.6 to 14 percent.

Intermittent fasting helps you eat less, and burn more calories. It promotes weight loss by switching up the regular calorie equation. It is also a good way to lose that bad belly fat that is often stored closely to organs which can cause diseases.

Remember the main reason this will help you lose weight is that you will be consuming fewer calories. If you consume an excessive amount of calories during the feeding windows of IF, then you're just making it harder for yourself to lose weight.

The body's ability to naturally burn fat is great, but it's not the only perk of trying intermittent fasting. Here are some more benefits to keep in mind:

- **This kind of fast will actually make your day easier.** You don't have to worry about getting up and making something to eat for breakfast. You can just grab your water or coffee and you're set. By cutting down the amount of meals you're having each day, you don't have to worry about spending all your time cooking, preparing and focusing on what you'll eat next. It just simplifies the day for you.

- **Intermittent fasting can help you live longer.** Studies have shown that restricting the amount of calories you take will lengthen your lifespan. When the body is in the fast state, it will find a way to sustain itself. The main problem here is that many people today eat so much food that they are not used to ever being in this fasting state. Therefor they are less willing to attempt it, even it it helps you live longer. The truth is fasting will activate all the same mechanisms that extend life just like calorie restriction.

- **Intermittent fasting can reduce the risk of cancer.** There was a study performed on ten cancer patients that proved that their chemo side effects diminished once they start fasting before their treatment. This occurred because they starved their cells clean of the sickness through the process of autophagy. Fasting also helps to reduce the risk of cardiovascular disease

- *Heart health*: IF can lower insulin resistance, inflammatory markers, blood sugar, blood triglycerides, and LDL cholesterol. These can all cause heart disease.

- *Inflammation*: Studies have shown a significant reduction of inflammation which are commonly the causes of many chronic diseases.

- *Insulin resistance*: IF helps to reduce the risk of insulin resistance and lowers blood sugar by about six percent with fasting levels by about 31 percent. This can help against preventing type 2 diabetes.

- *Brain health*: Fasting will raise the hormone BDNF and helps grow new nerve cells. It can also protect against Alzheimer's disease.

- *Weight loss*: IF significantly reduces your overall weight and belly fat, and you won't have to restrict your calories.

Putting all these health benefits aside, a lot of people have questions and concerns about intermittent fasting, especially if they're new to it. So I will now answer some of the most common questions about IF to help put your mind at ease:

- **Can I drink liquids while I'm fasting?** Yes absolutely! You can drink tea, coffee, water or other calorie-free beverages. Just make sure that whatever you drink is unsweetened.

- **Isn't not eating breakfast bad for you?** This is not
  true. Most stereotypical people who skip breakfast are
  people that don't eat healthy anyway. If you eat healthy
  foods throughout the day in your feeding windows you are
  going to be fine. You will start feeling and seeing the
  positive health changes happening regardless of having
  breakfast or not.

- **Is it alright to exercise in the fasted state?** Yes, you
  can exercise during the fasted state. In fact it is actually
  better for you to work out before eating. Just remember to
  not excessively exercise and over exert yourself.

- **Does fasting cause muscle loss?** Fasting does not
  directly cause muscle loss anymore so then any other
  method of weight loss. All forms of weight loss can cause
  you to lose muscle mass, so that's why lifting weights and
  eating lots of protein is encouraged. Intermittent fasting
  causes less muscle loss then restricting calories.

- **Does Fasting slow down your metabolsim?** No,
  intermittent fasting does not slow down your metabolism.
  In fact it will actually boost your metabolism. Only fasting
  for three consecutive days, meaning you don't eat anything
  for three whole days, can suppress metabolism. This length
  of fasting is not apart of intermittent fasting.

Now, there are some biological reactions that will occur within
your body while doing IF. Being hungry is the most difficult part.
At first, you may feel a little weak and that your brain isn't working
like normal. These will be temporary since your body will need
time to adapt to your new way of eating. If you're worried about
its impact on your health, then speak with your healthcare

provider before you start fasting.

Intermittent fasting isn't for everybody. If you have suffered from an eating disorder or are underweight, then this isn't something you should do without first consulting your doctor. It can cause more harm than good if your body is not in the right state.

You need to consult your doctor first before starting intermittent fasting if you are:

- Breastfeeding or pregnant.

- Female with a history of amenorrhea.

- Female trying to get pregnant.

- History of eating disorders.

- Underweight.

- Take prescription medications.

- Low blood pressure.

- Regulating blood sugar.

- Diabetes.

Although it's not for everyone, intermittent fasting does have a great safety profile. It isn't dangerous. You will be perfectly fine not eating for over 12 hours as long as you are moderately healthy, well nourished, and do not come under any of the points listed above.

Now as I have mentioned before in the introduction, this book primarily focuses on ketogenic diet recipes and meal plans that are made for your intermittent fasting feeding windows. As such my other books go much more in depth about explaining the details of intermittent fasting and preparing you with the knowledge needed before you start.

So if you want to know more information about intermittent fasting before starting, feel free to check out my other two books:

- <u>Intermittent Fasting For Women: Beat The Food Craving, And Get That Weight Shaving</u>

- <u>Intermittent Fasting: The Uncovered Celebrity Secret To Accelerate Weight Loss, Build Lean Muscle Fast, And Secure Your Healthiest Body And Mind</u>

If the links do not work, for whatever reason, you can simply search for these titles on the Amazon website to find them. Alternatively, you can visit my author page on Amazon to find these books.

What is the Ketogenic Diet?

The ketogenic diet is a low-carb, high-fat diet that has many health benefits for anyone who decides to undergo this lifestyle change. This diet can help you improve your health and lose significant weight. It has also been shown that a keto diet can help with Alzheimer's disease, epilepsy, cancer, and diabetes.

As the diet is high in fat and low in carbs, it has similarities to other low-carb diets like the Atkins diet. The keto diet primarily involves reducing your carb consumption and adding in fat. Reducing the amount of carbs you take will cause your body to enter a state called 'ketosis'. When you get into ketosis, your body begins to burn fat for energy instead of carbs. It will turn fat in the liver into ketones that give energy to the brain. In addition to this the keto diet can also greatly reduce insulin and blood sugar levels.

There are different types of the ketogenic diet:

- High protein: This is fairly similar to the standard but allows you to eat more protein. The ratio is typically 5% carbs, 60% fat, and 35% protein.

- Targeted (TKD): This lets you eat carbs before and after workouts.

- Cyclical (CKD): This is where you cycle high and low-carb days. For example you can eat the low-carb ketogenic way for five days, followed by two days where you eat larger amounts of carbs.

- Standard (SKD): This is the typical keto diet. It consists of 5% carbs, 75% fat, and 20% protein.

The standard and high protein diets have had many studies done on them and are typically the most popular. Targeted or cyclical diets are typically used more by bodybuilders or athletes.

The keto diet is a perfect way to lose weight and to reduce your risk for diseases. Studies have shown that the keto diet is much better for you than the recommended low-fat diet. There are many reasons for this, however the main contributing factor is the improved protein intake that will give you much more health benefits. This diet also helps you to feel full, and you won't have to count your calories or track your food as much.

Studies have shown that people who partook in a keto diet lost 2.2 times more weight than people who were on a low-calorie diet. HDL cholesterol and triglyceride levels also got significantly better. In addition to this the ketogenic dieters lost three times more weight than the people who ate a recommended diabetes diet.

Let's now get into what happens within your body during the keto diet. The keto in the ketogenic diet is because the body produces ketones. This is what the body uses for energy when glucose levels are low. Ketones get produced when you don't consume many carbs, and protein intake stays moderate. More ketones will help to improve insulin sensitivity and lower blood sugar levels. Too high of a protein level can increase blood sugar.

The liver makes the ketones from stored fat. This helps to fuel the entire body, which includes the brain. The brain demands a lot of energy each day. While on this diet, the body will switch its energy supply almost entirely to fat. Insulin drops and fat burning improves. This is perfect for when you want to lose weight, not to mention the steady amount of energy you get. This also becomes easier for you as your not as hungry anymore.

As I mentioned earlier when the body begins to produce ketones, it is called being in the state of 'ketosis'. The fastest way to actually reach this state is with fasting. However you can't fast forever, there will be times when it is healthier to eat something. This is why combining intermittent fasting with the ketogenic diet during your feeding windows, is the ultimate burning fat combination. They both compliment each other as they are both geared towards getting your body to produce ketones and entering the state of ketosis.

A keto diet is safe for many, but if you have the following situations, you might need more support by consulting your doctor:

- You are taking insulin for diabetes.

- You are taking medication for high blood pressure.

- You are breastfeeding.

What can you eat on a ketogenic diet?

You need to base most of your meals around these:

- Condiments: Spices, Herbs, pepper, and salt.

- Low-carb veggies: Peppers, onions, tomatoes, any green vegetable.

- Avocados: Whole or guacamole.

- Healthy oils: Mostly coconut oil, avocado oil, and extra virgin olive oil.

- Seeds and nuts: Chia seeds, pumpkin seeds, flax seeds, walnuts, almonds, etc.

- Cheese: Any unprocessed cheese like mozzarella, blue,

cream, goat, cheddar, etc.

- Cream and butter: Try to find grass fed if at all possible.

- Eggs: Look for Omega-3 whole eggs or free range.

- Fatty fish: Mackerel, tuna, trout, and salmon.

- Meat: Turkey, chicken, bacon, sausage, ham, steak, red meat.

The most important thing to help you reach ketosis is to stay away from carbs. You will need to keep your daily carbohydrate intake under 25 grams if you want to lose a significant amount of weight fast, or under 50 grams if you want to be more flexible.

What should you not eat on a ketogenic diet?

- Sugary foods: candy, ice cream, cake, smoothies, fruit juice, soda, etc.

- Starches and grains: cereal, pasta, rice, wheat-based products, etc.

- Fruit: all fruits except berries.

- Legumes and beans: chickpeas, lentils, kidney beans, peas, etc.

- Tubers and root vegetables: Parsnips, carrots, sweet potatoes, potatoes, etc.

- Some sauces and condiments: Look at the label. Some have unhealthy fats and sugars.

- Anything that is way too high in carbs for your daily intake

Remember to follow a very low-carb diet that is high in fat and moderate in protein.

What are you allowed to drink while on a keto diet? Water is best. Tea and coffee are okay as long as they are unsweet. Using cream or milk is fine. An occasional glass of wine is allowed too. Make sure to check the amount of carbs on other drinks such as beer and cider, as they are usually much more carb heavy.

If you find yourself needing a snack, here are some healthy snack ideas:

- Celery with guacamole and salsa.

- Strawberries and cream.

- Full-fat yogurt mixed with cocoa powder and nut butter.

- Low-carb milkshakes with nut butter, cocoa powder, and almond milk.

- 90% dark chocolate.

- 1 to 2 hard-boiled eggs.

- Olives with cheese.

- A handful of seeds or nuts.

- Cheese.

- Fish or fatty meat.

- Small portions of leftovers.

Why Choose the Ketogenic Diet?

I will now list the multitude of health benefits that come with this diet and why you should consider this diet for your new daily eating rituals.

Lose Weight

The most prominent benefit is turning your body into a fat burning machine that burns your fat away automatically to give you more energy. By automatically I mean you don't even have to exercise and yet your body will still burn the fat away for you. The rate of this burning fat is also increased whenever your insulin levels drop drastically. This creates the perfect conditions for fat loss to happen without being hungry.

Low-carb and ketogenic diets are more effective then others when trying to lose weight.

Reversal of Type 2 Diabetes

This diet can reverse type 2 diabetes because blood sugar levels are lowered and it impacts high insulin levels. Studies have shown that the ketogenic diet improves insulin sensitivity by 75 percent.

Other studies showed that some diabetes patients were able to stop their medication. In another study, a keto group lost 24.4 pounds as compared to 15.2 in a high-carb group. This is beneficial when you think about the connection between type 2 diabetes and weight.

About 95.2% of the group of keto dieters were able to reduce or stop their medications as opposed to the 62% of the high-carb dieters.

Better Mental Focus

The brain will get a steady flow of ketones. With a ketogenic diet, you stay away from large swings in blood sugar. This causes increased focus and better concentration.

Many people use keto for the increased mental performance. There is a misconception around that consuming many carbs is what the brain needs to function properly. This is false information and would only true if there are were no ketones available. However that is not the case with the ketogenic diet as there are plenty of ketones available and further more when in the state of ketosis.

After about a week of getting used to the keto diet, the brain and body run great on ketones. While in this state, many will experience improved mental focus and more energy. During the transition time, some might experience problems concentrating, being irritated, and having headaches. This is a natural occurrence as the body is just trying to adapt to a new way of living.

Better Physical Endurance

Keto diets can increase your physical endurance and provide you with constant energy by having access to your fat stores. The supply of stored carbohydrates in your body could only last for a couple hours of intense exercise. Comparatively, the stored fat could carry the energy you need for weeks, maybe even months.

If your body has adapted to only burning carbs because of all the high carb meals you eat throughout the day, then your fat stores aren't available and aren't able to fuel the brain. This means you would have to eat before, possibly during, and after exercising. Or you would have eat like that just to fuel the body to do your daily chores and stop being hungry all the time.

With this diet, that problem goes away. The brain and body are fueled easily by all the fat that has been stored, so you can just keep on going. Make sure to consume plenty of salt and fluids and to allow for keto-adaptation.

Metabolic Syndrome

Many studies have been done that show a low-carb diet can help the markers of metabolic syndrome like fasting blood sugar levels, LDL particle size, HDL-cholesterol, insulin levels, and blood lipids. The improvements are even greater when protein and carbs are restricted to staying in a steady ketosis.

Alzheimer's Disease

It is possible to prevent Alzheimer's disease by limiting foods that increase insulin levels. Insulin resistance causes Alzheimer's in the brain. This basically starves the brain of energy and leads to cognitive malfunction.

It is possible that Alzheimer's can be reduced by following a ketogenic diet. It probably won't cure dementia, but it should improve the condition. The most powerful effect is that it could reduce the risk of developing Alzheimer's disease completely.

Polycystic Ovary Syndrome

PCOS is common and affects about ten percent of women in childbearing years. Beyond causing menstrual and other physical problems, it is the leading cause of infertility.

There is a lifestyle change that can help treat this.

Here are some symptoms of PCOS:

- Obesity

- Excessive body hair and facial hair

- Acne

- Infertility

- Menstrual problems like heavy, skipped, or irregular periods.

PCOS is most common in women who are overweight, have type 2 diabetes, have excess insulin, or insulin resistance. Due to the connection of excess weight, other metabolic problems and high insulin levels, a low-carb diet is a great solution to help reverse PCOS. The ketogenic diet is the only treatment that will constantly lower insulin levels and reverses metabolic issues like PCOS. A low-carb diet needs to be at the center of any treatment meant for PCOS. Doctors who have used a low-carb diet to treat PCOS, support this as a great treatment for PCOS.

Ketosis

How am I going to know I'm in ketosis? You can find ketone levels by testing the urine, breath, or blood. Some symptoms require no testing:

- Increased Energy: After the beginning transition period of the 'keto flu' has passed, many experience much better energy. You can feel this as a sense of euphoria, no more brain fog, and clearer thinking.

- Reduced Hunger: Most won't feel as hungry. This could be due to the body switching over to using stored fat. Most people can get by with eating fewer meals. This saves money and time, and speeds up the weight loss process.

- Keto Breath: There is a ketone body known as acetone that leaves the body through our breath. It makes the breath smell like polish remover or fruity. This can be smelled when sweating as well. This is just a temporary side effect.

- Increased Urination: A different ketone body, acetoacetate, goes to the urine. This is why you can test for ketosis by using urine strips. When beginning a keto diet, it results in having to use the bathroom a lot. This is why you will experience an increased thirst.

- Increased Thirst and Dry Mouth: If you don't consume enough salt and water, you may end up with a dry mouth. You could start drinking a cup or two of bouillon each day. The main thing to remember here is to always drink plenty of water.

Getting into ketosis isn't black or white. It's not as if you are in or out of ketosis. There are several ketosis degrees and a lot of things that can increase your ketosis level.

1. You could restrict carbs even further to just 20 grams each day or less. Fiber isn't counted in this.

2. Keep protein moderate. You should consume one gram of protein per kg of your weight each day. It would be beneficial to lower protein if you are overweight. The mistake most people make is eating too much protein.

3. Consume fat to help feel full. This is what keeps the keto diet from ever causing you to starve. Keto diets are sustainable; starving isn't.

4. Stay away from snacks. Unnecessary snacking will slow down weight loss and reduce ketosis.

5. Exercise. Adding any type of physical activity will help to reverse type 2 diabetes and speed up weight loss.

What makes the keto diet even more enjoyable and simple, is that you don't need to learn any new skills. You might be wondering how to cook keto breakfasts that are tasty? How to consume more fat? What to do when dining out?

Here are some brief guidelines to follow, as the actual recipes are mentioned later:

Breakfast

Breakfast is a great time to incorporate a keto diet. You get to eat bacon and eggs. Another option is just to have coffee since some are not as hungry on a keto diet and don't' need breakfast. This will save you a lot of time.

Lunch & Dinner

What are you going to fix for lunch and dinner? You could have chicken, fish, or red meat with vegetables and a rich, full-fat cheesy sauce.

Dining Out

How can I eat keto at buffets, fast-food restaurants, or at a friend's house? Most offer meat or fish-based dishes. Ask for vegetables instead of high-carb foods. Egg-based meals like bacon and eggs or omelets are good options. Most fast food places offer bun-less burgers. At Mexican places, enjoy any meat with cheese, sour cream, salsa, and guacamole. For dessert ask for double cream and berries or a mixed cheese board.

Bread

If you just can't live without bread, there are bad and good options out there. The most important thing to do is to check the label for carbs under 6 net grams per serving. There are some great ones out there but generally speaking you want to avoid bread and when dining out just eat what's inside of it instead.

Eat More Fat

Fat is filling and enhances flavors. You should eat enough to make you feel full instead of hungry.

Stay Away from Special Products

A common mistake of new keto dieters is being fooled by the marketing hype of low-carb products. Effective dieting is based on real not processed foods. Low-carb products like bread, pasta, candy, and chocolate use deceptive marketing to make you think it is healthy when it is nothing more than just junk food in disguise.

Side Effects of Ketosis

If you completely cut out all starches and sugar, you could experience some side effects until your body becomes adjusted. These are usually mild and last only a few days. There are ways to lessen them.

Decreasing your intake of carbs slowly will help to minimize the side effects. Completely doing it is best for most. Removing starch and sugar usually results in several pounds lost within a few days. This will be mostly fluids, but it's a great motivator.

The most common side effect of starting a keto diet is the keto flu. This is what makes some people feel bad for about three days after beginning the diet. The symptoms are:

- Irritability

- Light nausea

- Dizziness

- Fatigue

- Headache

These will go away as your body becomes adjusted and the fat burning increases. They usually last only a week at max.

Foods that are rich in carbs cause water retention. When you stop eating these foods, you will lose excess salt and water through the kidneys and this will cause you to pee more than normal. This could result in dehydration and lack of salt in the first week.

You can minimize the effects of the keto flu by drinking lots of water and increasing your salt intake.

Keto Myths

There are many fears and myths out there that just don't hold true under close scrutiny. The funniest one is that your brain won't work if you don't eat carbs. This is simply not true.

Another mistake is mixing up ketosis with the medical emergency ketoacidosis. These are two entirely different things. Ketoacidosis can't happen just from eating a keto diet.

Ketoacidosis is a dangerous and rare condition that can happen to type 1 diabetics if they don't get enough insulin.

Ketosis is a natural and safe state that is controlled by the body. It can be caused by a period of fasting or a low-carb diet.

Under normal circumstances, a strict low-carb diet will never result in ketoacidosis. It results in ketosis and a natural state that allows the body to burn large amounts of fat.

I can assure you from experience that any fears people have about the ketogenic diet are just purely based on misunderstandings.

Supplements

Supplements are generally not needed, but some might be useful. If you find yourself in need, here are some to consider:

- Whey: Use half a scoop in yogurt and shakes to increase protein intake.

- Creatine: This provides many benefits for performance and health. This will help if you combine exercise and the ketogenic diet.

- Exogenous ketones: This may raise your ketone levels.

- Caffeine: This gives the benefits of performance, fat loss, and energy.

- Minerals: Added minerals and salt is important when beginning because of shifts in mineral balance and water.

- MCT Oil: Add this to yogurt and drinks. It provides energy and can help to increase ketone levels.

Just like any diet, keto only works if you stick with it. But if I was to recommend any diet pattern to you where you have to eat certain types of food, it would be the ketogenic diet every time.

The Ketogenic Diet with Intermittent Fasting

Intermittent fasting and the ketogenic diet are both hot topics that often fall into conversations these days, especially in the health and fitness industry. Some differences make you wonder if one is better than the other, or if they can both fit into your life.

Let's now compare intermittent fasting and the ketogenic diet. We've already covered what each one does in the previous chapters, so let's see some brief similarities and differences that they share. Afterwards we will discuss some important tips on how to intermittent fast on the ketogenic diet.

Similarities

Ketosis is a direct result of starving the body of either carbs or food in general. This is why the ketogenic diet and intermittent fasting have much of the same benefits. They work with each other very well as they are aiming towards the same goal, entering and maintaining ketosis.

Just like the ketogenic diet, intermittent fasting involves times of starving the body of either carbs or food. However because you are still eating food on the ketogenic diet, intermittent fasting actually gets the body into ketosis faster, because you're having no carbs or food at all when you're in the fasting state.

If you look at intermittent fasting and the ketogenic diet, you can see that each one complements the other. Both have benefits for weight loss and health, and that has more to do with fasting than ketosis.

Differences

The most obvious and main difference is, one involves eating while the other doesn't. You can eat throughout the day and stay in ketosis when doing the ketogenic diet. Whereas intermittent fasting means you won't eat any food for a certain amount of time.

The ketogenic diet's goal is to put your body into ketosis. Intermittent fasting isn't a diet and just because you choose to do it, doesn't mean your goal is to be in ketosis. Some intermittent fast just to eat less during the day and to keep from overeating at night. Somebody might choose to do a keto diet for more than just to lose weight.

Important advice for trying to intermittent fast on the ketogenic diet:

1. Don't try to intermittent fast in the first two weeks of starting the ketogenic diet or if you follow the Standard American Diet. This is extremely important. Your body needs to get adapted to the keto diet before you try intermittent fasting. Your body must get used to eating low-carbs so your body can utilize ketones for energy instead of using glucose. If you try intermittent fasting at the same time you begin the keto diet, you will not succeed. You will be too glucose-dependent and too hungry to stick with it. There is some misinformation around about intermittent fasting. Intermittent fasting needs to be natural and not a struggle, and you should never feel hungry. It will be a gradual process and take time before it is used effectively.

2. Don't try to plan intermittent fasting too much. You must listen to your body. Intermittent fasting works best if it is done naturally. If you realize it's lunchtime, but you don't feel hungry, just skip it and eat at dinner time. If it is too late to eat? Skip dinner and eat breakfast. Most people find

it easier to skip breakfast anyway. Try to eat about 1 pm, and eat again about four hours before you go to bed, so your body has time to digest your foods.

3. Start slow. Don't force yourself to do the complete intermittent fasting schedule immediately. You should never deprive or restrict yourself. When your body has become fat-adapted, you won't feel as hungry. Begin by staying away from snacks between meals. Next, try skipping regular meals. Do this only if you don't feel hungry.

4. Stay busy. You might find it easier to skip meals if you are busy and don't spend time in the kitchen. You might be tempted to have a snack if you are around food, even if you don't feel hungry. It is easy to go without food when you are out shopping. Remember to drink plenty of liquid. Water, tea, or coffee is all you need.

5. Intermittent fasting is just one tool to help you reach your goal. It helps with weight loss, longevity, and many other things, but it is just one factor that helps you meet your target. Exercise, micronutrients, macronutrients, sufficient sleep, and stress levels are some things to consider. Never use intermittent fasting as a quick fix when you have overindulged.

6. Butter or bulletproof coffee will break your fasting. Eating coconut oil or butter will not keep you in a fasted state. Anything that has calories will have the same effect. That's why it is called fasting. If you must have coffee in the mornings, add some cream but skip the sugar, butter, and oils.

7. Remember as I mentioned earlier, intermittent fasting isn't for everyone. If you come under any of the conditions below

you should not do intermittent fasting:

- Type 1 diabetes

- Type 2 diabetics should only do it under a doctor's supervision since they might need to adjust their medication.

- Bulimia nervosa

- Anorexia nervosa

- Adrenal or chronic fatigue disorders

- Breastfeeding

- Pregnant women

- Very stressed

- Exercise too much

- Don't get enough sleep

If you have any side effects such as hormone imbalance, irregular periods, anxiety, or sleeplessness, you should consult your health care practitioner before continuing.

The Different Intermittent Fasting Methods

In the next few chapters, you will find lots of ketogenic recipes to use in your meal plans for your intermittent fasting eating windows. They will contain all of the macro information that you need to keep track of. First, we will look at the different intermittent fasting cycles so that you can understand which keto recipes to use.

This will also help you to pick a cycle that works best for you. If you're going to have to force yourself to follow a method, then chances are it's not going to well for you. Pick the method that will make your life easier, and you will be able to follow it.

Each of these cycles will have its own rules for the length that you fast, and what you should eat during the feeding phase. Will look at some of the most popular fasting methods and how they work.

For all of these, you will need to figure out your own macros that suit you. Not everybody is going to have the same macros they can consume each day.

Lean gains

This cycle is best for the dedicated gym-goers who are interested in burning body fat and building muscle.

For a woman, you fast for 14 hours, and for a man, you fast for 16 hours every day. You eat during the remaining eight to ten hours. While fasting, you cannot have any calories. You can, however, have sugar-free gum, diet soda, calorie-free sweeteners, and black coffee. If you need to, you can add a splash of milk to your coffee. Most people who follow this will fast through the night and into the morning. The fast is typically broken around six hours after waking. This can be easily adapted to anybody's schedule; the most important thing is maintaining a consistent feeding window. Otherwise, hormones can get messed up and causes the program to be a lot harder.

The things that you eat and when you eat will also depend on when you exercise. The days that you exercise, you may need a bit more carbs than fat. On the days that you rest, consuming more fats is preferable. Protein consumption should be at a steady intake every day, though the amount will vary based on your activity level, body fat, age, gender, and goals. Regardless of what diets you choose to follow, you should consume whole, unprocessed foods. 50-60% of your calories need to be eaten after your workout.

The pros of this are that during your eight-hour feeding window, you can eat whenever you want. Meal frequency doesn't really play a factor in this. Some people will find it easier if they do break it up into three meals though.

The cons are that even though it has the flexibility of choosing when to eat, lean gains does have a very specific guideline of the foods that you can eat, especially when it comes to working out. Sticking to the nutrition plan and scheduling your meals around exercising all the time can make this be harder to stick to.

A typical day could look like:

Monday:

- Breakfast 12:00 pm – 1:00 pm

- Lunch 4:00 pm – 5:00 pm

- Dinner 8:00 pm – 9:00 pm

- *Fasting:* Monday 9:00 pm – Tuesday 12:00 pm

Eat Stop Eat

This fasting cycle works for healthy eaters that need a little extra boost.

For this cycle, you will fast for 24 hours once or twice each week. Some people will refer to the 24-hour fast time as a 24-hour break from eating. You aren't allowed to consume any food during this time, but you can have calorie-free beverages. Once the 24 hours are up, you can go back to eating like you normally would. There are some people that may want to end the 24 hours with a big dinner meal, and others are okay with just having a snack.

The main reason behind this fasting cycle is to reduce your overall calorie intake without having to limit the foods that you eat. Having a regular workout routine helps, especially resistance training. This will up your weight loss and improve your body composition.

The pros of this cycle are that even though 24 hours may seem like a really long time to go without eating, the program is flexible. You don't have to be perfect when you first start out. Go as many hours as you can on the first day and then start upping the time you fast so that your body can adjust. It's best if you start your first fasting time on a day where you don't have any eating obligations and a day where you are busy so that your mind is distracted.

Another pro is that there aren't any forbidden foods, and you don't have count calories. This makes it a bit easier to follow. But this shouldn't just be a free-for-all. You should eat responsibly and choose healthy options. The healthiest option would still be to combine your eating days with the ketogenic diet.

The main con is going for a 24 hours fast without any calories can be hard for some at the beginning. A lot of people complain about experiencing anxiety, crankiness, fatigue, or headaches. These side effects will go away once your system gets used to it. It can also sometimes be more tempting to binge once your fasting time is over. You will need some self-control to fix this problem.

A typical meal plan would look like:

Friday:

- Breakfast 7 – 8 am

- Lunch 12 – 1 pm

- Dinner 5 – 7 pm

Fasting:

- Friday 7 pm – Saturday 7 pm

Saturday:

- Dinner 7 pm – 8 pm

You would then eat normally for the rest of the week until 7 pm Friday, or you could add another fast in from 7 pm Monday to 7 pm Tuesday.

5:2 Diet

The 5:2 diet gets its name from the fact that five days out of the week you eat like normal and the other two days will restrict your calories down to 500-600 a day. This plan by itself doesn't actually restrict the foods that you eat, but instead when to eat them. This makes it a lot easier to stick to for a lot of people as opposed to counting calories.

You can pick whatever two days you fast, as long as there is an eating day in between them. The most common plan is to fast on Mondays and Thursdays and eat a couple of little meals, and then eat normally for the remainder of the week. Make sure that you don't binge eat on your eating days.

For this one, you actually eat on fasting days just smaller meals that fit into the 500-600 calorie range. The meals you eat should be high-fiber foods that will help you to feel fuller without needing the extra calories.

The downside is that during the first few days you may experience extreme hunger, and you may feel slow or weak. Once your body gets used to it, these problems will go away. During the first week or so you can keep yourself busy so that you don't have time to think about it. If you start to feel ill though, you need to make sure you have something to eat like a salad.

A typical meal plan would look something like:

Monday (fast day)

- Breakfast 7 – 8 am 130 calories

- Lunch 12 – 1 pm 180 calories

- Dinner 5 – 6 pm 190 calories

Tuesday (normal)

Wednesday (normal)

Thursday (fast day)

- Breakfast 7 – 8 am 130 calories

- Lunch 12 – 1 pm 180 calories

- Dinner 5 – 6 pm 190 calories

Friday (normal)

Saturday (normal)

Sunday (normal)

Alternate-Day Fasting

This one is best for a disciplined dieter that has a goal weight in mind.

This one works similar to the 5:2 except you alternate low-calorie and normal calorie every day. On your low-cal, or fast day, you will eat a fifth of your typical calorie intake. If you go by the average 2,000 for women and 2,500 for men, you will consume 400-500 calories.

To help out on the fasting days, you can choose meal replacement shakes that fit into your diet. You can sip on them throughout the day while keeping your calories low. This will help trick your brain into thinking you are consuming more food than you actually are. They are also full of nutrients. This should only be used during the first two weeks while you are getting used to fasting. After that, you need to start consuming real foods on your fasting days. If you work out, you may notice on fast days that you feel weaker, so you should be more gentle to your body on those days.

The pros for this choice are that if your goal is to lose weight, then this is perfect for you. When a person cuts their calorie intake by 20-35 percent you will see a weight loss of about two and a half pounds each week.

The cons for this option are that while it may be easy to follow, it's also easy to overeat on a normal day. The best way to make sure that you follow through and don't overeat is to plan out your meals on the ketogenic diet. This way you won't be caught at a drive-through at some fast food restaurant.

A typical week would look like:

Sunday (normal)

Monday (fast)

- Breakfast 100 calories

- Lunch 150 calories

- Dinner 150 calories

Tuesday (normal)

Wednesday (fast)

- Breakfast 100 calories

- Lunch 150 calories

- Dinner 150 calories

Thursday (normal)

Friday (fast)

- Breakfast 100 calories

- Lunch 150 calories

- Dinner 150 calories

Saturday (normal)

16:8 Diet

This is one of the most popular fasting options, and probably the easiest to follow. This is similar to the lean gains method, but it doesn't have as strict rules on calorie intake. This is where you fast for 16 hours, typically overnight, and then eating the other eight hours. You can have a cup of coffee at breakfast and then eat your first meal at noon or one.

This is probably the best option for somebody following the ketogenic diet. It doesn't add any other rules that you have to follow, nor does it require strict exercise routines. You could choose to do this every day, or just do it a few times a week. Following a low-carb diet can sometimes cause you to start unconsciously following a 16:8 fasting cycle just because you don't feel as hungry.

A typical eating period would look like:

Monday:

- Breakfast 12:00 pm – 2:00 pm

- Lunch 4:00 pm – 5:00 pm

- Dinner 7:00 pm – 8:00 pm

- *Fasting:* Monday 8:00 pm – Tuesday 12:00 pm

Tuesday:

- Breakfast 12:00 pm – 2:00 pm

- Lunch 4:00 pm – 5:00 pm

- Dinner 7:00 pm – 8:00 pm

- *Fasting:* Tuesday 8:00 pm – Wednesday 12:00 pm

Ketogenic Recipes

Breakfast

Chili Cheese Muffins

Cook Time: 30 minutes   **Prep Time:** 15 minutes

Ingredients:

½ tsp baking soda

3 eggs

2 cups packed cheddar cheese

½ tsp salt

1 ¼ cup almond flour

Instructions:

You should set your oven to 350°F.

Combine the salt, baking soda, and flour in your food processor. Pulse the eggs until combined.

Add the cheese and a tablespoon of the pepper flakes. Add the batter to the muffin tin cups, about a quarter cup in each.

Sprinkle the tops with the remaining pepper flakes. Place in the oven for 25 to 30 minutes. Enjoy!

Servings: 12

Nutrition:

- **Calories:** 110
- **Net Carbs:** .5 g
- **Proteins:** 6.8 g
- **Fats:** 8.84 g

Porridge

Cook Time: 0 minutes   **Prep Time:** 15 minutes

Ingredients:

1 tbsp of each:

- flaxseed

- pumpkin seeds

- chia seeds

1 cup boiling water

1 tsp cinnamon

¼ cup walnuts

2 tbsp unsweetened coconut

¼ tsp sea salt

Instructions:

Use a food processor to mix all the dry ingredients until these are finely ground.

Start adding in the water and mix it up until it has become smooth.

Add the porridge to a bowl and top it off with some extra sunflower seeds or coconut.

Enjoy!

Servings: 1

Nutrition:

- **Calories:** 747
- **Net Carbs:** 9.27 g
- **Proteins:** 15.84 g
- **Fats:** 66.37 g

Jalapeno Popper Egg Cups

Cook Time: 25 minutes   **Prep Time:** 10 minutes

Ingredients:

Pepper and salt

½ tsp onion powder

4 oz cheddar cheese

½ tsp garlic powder

3 oz cream cheese

8 eggs

4 jalapenos, chopped

12 bacon strips

Instructions:

Your oven should be set to 375°F. Par-cook your bacon so that it is slightly crisp, but you can still move it. Keep the bacon greased.

With a hand mixer, beat everything together except for the one jalapeno and the cheddar.

Grease a muffin tin up and then wrap a slice of bacon around the edges of each cup.

Pour the eggs into the muffin tin, making sure not to overfill.

Sprinkle the cheddar over the top of each, and place a jalapeno ring into each of the cups.

Cook for 20 to 25 minutes. Enjoy!

Servings: 12

Nutrition:

- **Calories:** 157
- **Net Carbs:** 1.35 g
- **Proteins:** 9.75 g
- **Fats:** 12.28 g

Bacon and Cheese Cauliflower Muffins

Cook Time: 25 minutes   **Prep Time:** 15 minutes

Ingredients:

¼ cup feta cheese

Pepper and salt

2 eggs

1 tbsp of each:

- Parsley

- Paprika

- Garlic powder

- Oregano

7 slices chopped bacon

1 tsp baking powder

¼ cup almond flour

1 cup shredded cheese

3 cups cauliflower rice

Instructions:

Place the cauliflower in a bowl and mix in all the dry ingredients, cheese, and bacon.

Add the eggs and thoroughly mix them. You should be able to push the mixture with your spoon and it holds together.

Place your silicone muffin cups in a muffin tin.

Add the mixture in the cups and then top with the feta.

Your oven should be at 350°F.

Bake the muffins for 35 minutes. Enjoy!

Servings: 12

Nutrition:

- **Calories:** 109

- **Net Carbs:** 2.4 g

- **Proteins:** 6.62 g

- **Fats:** 7.98 g

Goat Cheese Tomato Tarts

Cook Time: 70 minutes   **Prep Time:** 25 minutes

Ingredients:

Tomatoes:

Pepper and salt

¼ cup olive oil

2 tomatoes, sliced

Base:

½ cup almond flour

5 tbsp cold butter, cubed

2 tbsp coconut flour

1 tbsp psyllium husk powder

¼ tsp salt

Filling:

3 oz goat cheese

3 tsp thyme

2 tsp minced garlic

2 tbsp olive oil

½ onion, sliced

Instructions:

Your oven should be at 435°F. Drizzle the tomato slices with oil and season with pepper and salt. Place the tomatoes into the oven for 40 minutes. Set to the side.

Turn the oven to 350°F. Use a food processor to mix all of the base ingredients.

Press the dough into 12 silicone cupcake molds. Place them in the oven for 20 minutes then take them out and allow to cool completely.

Gently remove the base from the molds.

Cook the garlic and onion in the olive oil until caramelized.

To complete the tart, place a tomato on the top with onion, thyme, and goat cheese. Do this to all of the bases. Bake them for six more minutes to melt the cheese.

Enjoy!

Servings: 12

Nutrition:

- **Calories:** 159

- **Net Carbs:** 1.57 g

- **Proteins:** 2.76 g

- **Fats:** 15.67 g

Italian Omelet

Cook Time: 10 minutes   **Prep Time:** 5 minutes

Ingredients:

2 eggs

2 oz mozzarella

1 tbsp water

5 slices tomato

1 tbsp butter

6 basil leaves

3 slices soppressata

Instructions:

Mix the eggs and the water. Add the butter to a skillet and allow it to melt. Pour the eggs and let them set for about 30 seconds.

Lay the meat onto half of the egg. Lay the basil, tomato, and cheese on top. Sprinkle everything with a bit of salt and pepper.

Continue to cook until the egg has set. Fold the other half of the egg over the ingredients. Place a lid over the skillet and let it cook for another two minutes.

Slide it out onto a plate and enjoy!

Servings: 1

Nutrition:

- **Calories:** 401

- **Net Carbs:** 5.4 g

- **Proteins:** 37.37 g

- **Fats:** 24.72 g

Sausage and Kale Hash

Cook Time: 30 minutes   **Prep Time:** 10 minutes

Ingredients:

7 oz kale

1 tsp Dijon mustard

2 minced garlic cloves

1 tbsp lemon juice

3 tbsp ghee

2 cups cauliflower, riced

5 oz sausage

Topping:

4 poached eggs

Instructions:

Place the cauliflower in your food processor and pulse it until it resembles rice. Remove the stalks from the kale and chop the kale.

Add a tablespoon of ghee to a skillet and add the sausage. Cook until the sausage is completely done and transfer it to a bowl.

Add the remaining ghee to the skillet then toss the garlic and sauté until it gives off fragrance. Add the riced cauliflower and let it cook for another five minutes. Make sure you often stir so that it doesn't burn.

Mix the kale, lemon juice, and Dijon, and let it cook for another two minutes. Add the salt and pepper to taste and stir everything together. Mix the kale and cook until the kale has softened.

Once done, mix the sausage back in, and then take it off the heat. Split the mixture between two plates and serve with poached eggs. Enjoy!

Servings: 2

Nutrition:

- **Calories:** 605

- **Net Carbs:** 7 g

- **Proteins:** 31.4 g

- **Fats:** 46.3 g

Brie and Bacon Frittata

Cook Time: 45 minutes   **Prep Time:** 10 minutes

Ingredients:

8 slices bacon

4 oz brie, sliced

8 eggs

½ tsp pepper

½ cup whipping cream

½ tsp salt

2 garlic cloves, minced

Instructions:

In a prepared skillet, cook the bacon slices until these become crispy. Drain the oil using the paper towel. Set the skillet off the heat, but keep the bacon grease in the pan.

Place two thirds of the crumbled bacon, cream, garlic, salt, pepper, and eggs in a bowl and whisk them all together. Set the skillet back on the heat and swirl the grease around to coat the pan.

Pour the eggs and let them cook. Do not touch the eggs. Allow it to cook until the edges have set and the center is still a bit loose. This takes about ten minutes.

In the meantime, turn on your broiler.

Set brie slices on the frittata and sprinkle the remaining bacon over the top.

Place the frittata in the oven and let it cook until it becomes puffy and golden. Make sure that it doesn't burn. This should take around ten more minutes.

Remove, and let it cool for a few minutes, and enjoy!

Servings: 4

Nutrition:

- **Calories:** 487

- **Net Carbs:** 2.2 g

- **Proteins:** 23.89 g

- **Fats:** 42.21 g

Lunch

Curried Shrimp

Cook Time: 20 minutes   **Prep Time:** 5 minutes

Ingredients:

4 tbsp olive oil

3 tbsp lime juice

4 garlic cloves

1 lb peeled shrimp

1 onion, chopped

Bunch Cilantro, chopped

½ cup tomatoes, pureed

½ tsp turmeric

2 tsp minced ginger

½ tsp coriander

½ tsp cumin

Instructions:

Add the oil to the skillet and cook the onions and garlic until they become soft. Stir the tomatoes, turmeric, ginger, coriander, and cumin.

Allow this to continue to cook for five more minutes. Add the shrimp and let the shrimp cook until it is cooked through and the shrimp turns pink.

Mix the lime juice and cilantro and enjoy!

Servings: 4

Nutrition:

- **Calories:** 267

- **Net Carbs:** 6 g

- **Proteins:** 24.42 g

- **Fats:** 15.26 g

Fish Sticks

Cook Time: 45 minutes   **Prep Time:** 15 minutes

Ingredients:

2 eggs, whisked

6 tbsp coconut oil

1 tsp salt

1 lb white fish

1 cup almond flour

Instructions:

Slice up your fish into sticks, making sure to get rid of any bones.

Combine the flour and the salt, and add the eggs to a separate bowl. Dip a fish stick in the eggs and then in the flour. Continue until all of the fish sticks have been coated.

Add half of the oil to a skillet and add half of the fish sticks. Cook until browned and fish is cooked through. Add the rest of the oil and cook the rest of the fish sticks. Enjoy!

Servings: 4

Nutrition:

- **Calories:** 523
- **Net Carbs:** 3.9 g
- **Proteins:** 31.28 g
- **Fats:** 43 g

Smoked Salmon and Goat Cheese Bites

Cook Time: 0 minutes   **Prep Time:** 25 minutes

Ingredients:

4 oz smoked salmon

3.9 oz radicchio

Salt and pepper

2 garlic cloves

1 tbsp basil

1 tbsp rosemary

1 tbsp oregano

8 oz goat cheese, softened

Instructions:

Finely mince up the basil, rosemary, and oregano. Grate the garlic. Place the pepper, garlic, salt, herbs, and goat cheese. Mix them all.

Slice the stem of the radicchio. Carefully take the leaves apart until you have 16. Wash and dry the leaves.

Place a piece of salmon on each leaf and top with the goat cheese mixture. Add a bit of pepper over the top of each. Enjoy!

Servings: 16

Nutrition:

- **Calories:** 46

- **Net Carbs:** .9 g

- **Proteins:** 3.43 g

- **Fats:** 3.33 g

Feta and Bacon Bites

Cook Time: 15 minutes   **Prep Time:** 10 minutes

Ingredients:

Salt and pepper

3 tbsp sriracha mayo

¼ cup chopped green onions

¼ cup feta cheese

8 bacon slices, cooked

2 cups mozzarella, shredded

¾ cup almond flour

Instructions:

You should have your oven at 350°F.

Heat a nonstick skillet and cook the mozzarella and almond flour together. Stir constantly. It should be dough consistency within five minutes.

Place this between two pieces of parchment and roll it out. Use a cookie cutter to make 24 circles.

Place this into a muffin tin and top with onion, feta, and bacon. Bake this for 15 minutes.

Peel off the liner and add some mayo on top. Enjoy!

Servings: 24

Nutrition:

- **Calories:** 71.79
- **Net Carbs:** 1.08 g
- **Proteins:** 3.66 g
- **Fats:** 5.74 g

Kale Chips

Cook Time: 12 minutes   **Prep Time:** 10 minutes

Ingredients:

1 tbsp seasoned salt

2 tbsp olive oil

1 large bunch kale

Instructions:

Your oven should be set to 350°F.

Take the stems off the kale and then wash and dry. Rip the kale up and place in a bag with the oil and shake so that the kale is coated.

Place the kale on a cookie sheet and spread them out. Cook for 12 minutes and then sprinkle with seasoned salt.

Enjoy!

Servings: 1

Nutrition:

- **Calories:** 80.5
- **Net Carbs:** 1.29 g
- **Proteins:** 1.82 g
- **Fats:** 7.15 g

Thai Chicken Wraps

Cook Time: 0 minutes   **Prep Time:** 20 minutes

Ingredients:

1 cup shredded carrots

Peanut sauce

12 romaine leaves

¼ cup sliced scallions

4 cabbage leaves, chopped

1 cup chopped broccoli

1 lb grilled chicken breast, diced

Instructions:

Mix the grilled diced chicken, broccoli, carrots, scallions, and cabbage together in a bowl.

Split the mixture between each of the romaine leaves.

Drizzle the top with some peanut sauce.

Enjoy!

Servings: 6

Nutrition:

- **Calories:** 261
- **Net Carbs:** 6 g
- **Proteins:** 29.5 g
- **Fats:** 11.05 g

Salmon Burgers

Cook Time: 20 minutes   **Prep Time:** 10 minutes

Ingredients:

1 lb salmon

1 tbsp coconut flour

1 tbsp sesame oil

2 eggs

1 tbsp ume plum vinegar

¼ cup sesame seeds

1 minced garlic clove

¼ cup chopped scallions

1 tsp minced ginger

Instructions:

Dice the salmon up into cubes and then stir in the oil, scallions, eggs, sesame seeds, ginger, garlic, and vinegar.

Follow with coconut flour.

Form the mixture into patties after splitting it into fourths.

Fry the patties in a skillet until they turn golden on both sides and the fish is cooked through.

Enjoy!

Servings: 4

Nutrition:

- **Calories:** 275
- **Net Carbs:** 1.2 g
- **Proteins:** 28.14 g
- **Fats:** 16.61 g

Meatballs

Cook Time: 25 minutes   **Prep Time:** 20 minutes

Ingredients:

1 tbsp coconut flour

¼ tsp baking soda

1 lb ground beef

2 tbsp Dijon

½ tsp sea salt

2 tbsp tomato paste

1 Egg

Shallot, minced

½ tsp pepper

Instructions:

Stir together the egg, shallot, and beef.

Mix all of the other ingredients.

Take a quarter cup of the mixture and form it into balls.

Set the meatballs onto a baking sheet. Continue until you have used up all the mixture.

You should set your oven to 350°F.

Place the meatballs into the oven and cook for 25 minutes. Enjoy!

Servings: 6

Nutrition:

- **Calories:** 418
- **Net Carbs:** 5.3 g
- **Proteins:** 22.82 g
- **Fats:** 31.46 g

Dinner

Beef Brisket

Cook Time: 8 hours   **Prep Time:** 5 minutes

Ingredients:

1 ½ lb brisket

½ tsp salt

1 tbsp onion powder

8 carrots, sliced

3 cup chicken stock

8 oz mushrooms, sliced

1 onion, chopped

8 sliced garlic cloves

1 tbsp garlic powder

Instructions:

Place everything, except for the brisket, into your slow cooker.

Mix all of the ingredients together.

Place the brisket into the mixture and place the lid on.

Set the cooker to low for eight hours. Enjoy!

Servings: 6

Nutrition:

- **Calories:** 225
- **Net Carbs:** 5 g
- **Proteins:** 29.42 g
- **Fats:** 7.43 g

Stir Fry

Cook Time: 40 minutes   **Prep Time:** 15 minutes

Ingredients:

1 lb chicken breast

2 tbsp ume plum vinegar

2 tbsp coconut oil

2 tbsp sesame oil

1 onion, chopped

2 tbsp arrowroot powder

2 heads broccoli

1 ½ cup water

2 carrots, sliced

½ tsp salt

2 heads bok choy, sliced

1 zucchini, sliced

4 oz shiitake, sliced

Instructions:

Cut the chicken into cubes. Add the coconut oil to a skillet and allow it to melt.

Add the onion and cook until it has become soft.

Stir in the carrots, chicken, and broccoli. Allow this mixture to cook for another ten minutes.

Stir in the bok choy, salt, mushrooms, and zucchini. Let this cook for an extra five minutes.

Add a cup of water and place a lid on the pan then allow this to cook for ten minutes.

Mix the arrowroot with a half cup of water.

Stir the mixture into the pan. Continue to stir and cook until it has all thickened.

Mix in the sesame oil and the vinegar. Enjoy!

Servings: 6

Nutrition:

- **Calories:** 366
- **Net Carbs:** 7.3 g
- **Proteins:** 23 g
- **Fats:** 17 g

Chicken and Cauliflower

Cook Time: 55 minutes   **Prep Time:** 60 minutes

Ingredients:

3 tbsp olive oil

5 sliced garlic cloves

Bunch of fresh thyme

1 lemon, zest

1 head cauliflower, florets

½ tsp salt

1 shallot, chopped

1 cup black olives

1 lb chicken breast

¼ cup lemon juice

1 tsp pepper

Instructions:

On the bottom of a casserole dish, lay the thyme then put the chicken on top and add the cauliflower over the chicken.

Mix all the remaining ingredients and pour it over the chicken. Allow this to sit and marinate for around an hour

You should place your oven to 400°F.

Place the chicken in your oven and cook for 45 to 55 minutes until chicken is cooked through. Enjoy!

Servings: 2

Nutrition:

- **Calories:** 581
- **Net Carbs:** 7.3 g
- **Proteins:** 57.82 g
- **Fats:** 32.6 g

Shepherd's Pie

Cook Time: 30 minutes   **Prep Time:** 20 minutes

Ingredients:

1 cup chicken stock

1 lb ground beef

1 lb diced turkey bacon

2 heads cauliflower, steamed

2 cups diced celery

2 cups diced carrots

½ tsp paprika

2 tbsp olive oil

1 tsp pepper

1 onion, diced

½ tsp salt

Instructions:

In your prepared pan, heat up the olive oil then toss the onion and sauté until soft. Stir in the bacon and let it cook until it is crisp. Mix in the carrots and celery. Cook until the vegetables become soft.

Add in the beef and let it cook until brown. Season the mixture with pepper, paprika, and salt. Add the broth and let the mixture reduce by about half.

Add the cauliflower and the remaining olive oil to a food processor and mix until it is smooth.

Add the beef mixture to a baking dish and top with the pureed cauliflower. You should set your oven to 350°F.

Place this into the oven for 30 minutes, and then enjoy!

Servings: 4

Nutrition:

- **Calories:** 760
- **Net Carbs:** 11 g
- **Proteins:** 68.67 g
- **Fats:** 77 g

Fried Mac and Cheese

Cook Time: 45 minutes   **Prep Time:** 15 minutes

Ingredients:

¾ tsp rosemary

1 tsp turmeric

2 tsp paprika

3 eggs

1 ½ c cheddar cheese

1 cauliflower head, riced

Instructions:

Microwave the riced cauliflower for five minutes and ring the water out with kitchen towels.

Mix the eggs into the riced cauliflower one at a time, then the cheese and spices.

Form this mixture into patties.

Heat some oil in a skillet.

Fry them in the skillet until browned and each side. Enjoy!

Servings: 12

Nutrition:

- **Calories:** 70
- **Net Carbs:** 1.8 g
- **Proteins:** 4.5 g
- **Fats:** 4.71 g

Spiced Bacon Deviled Eggs

Cook Time: 0 minutes   **Prep Time:** 15 minutes

Ingredients:

½ tsp rosemary

¼ tsp cayenne

1 tsp Dijon

1 tbsp bacon fat

2 slices bacon

¼ cup mayo

5 hard boiled eggs

Instructions:

Crumble up your cooked bacon, and slice the eggs in half.

Remove the yolks into a bowl.

Mix half of the rosemary, the bacon fat, cayenne, Dijon, and mayo.

Place some pieces of bacon into the bottom of each egg. Pipe the yolk mixture in each of the eggs and top with the rest of the bacon and rosemary.

Enjoy!

Servings: 3

Nutrition:

- **Calories:** 315

- **Net Carbs:** .8 g

- **Proteins:** 12.6 g

- **Fats:** 28 g

Pizza Chips

Cook Time: 15 minutes   **Prep Time:** 10 minutes

Ingredients:

5.25 oz shredded mozzarella

6 oz pepperoni, sliced

Instructions:

Your oven should be placed on 400°F.

Arrange the pepperoni in batches of four.

Layer the pepperoni on top of each other and place onto a baking sheet.

Place this into the oven for about five minutes.

Take the pizza chips out of the oven and sprinkle the cheese on each of them.

Then bake for another three minutes.

Set the chips on paper towels to soak up the grease, and enjoy!

Servings: 21

Nutrition:

- **Calories:** 61.29
- **Net Carbs:** .16 g
- **Proteins:** 3 g
- **Fats:** 5.3 g

Turkey Stuffed Peppers

Cook Time: 60 minutes **Prep Time:** 20 minutes

Ingredients:

1 tbsp olive oil

1 tsp chili powder

1 tsp salt

6 bell peppers

1 cup chopped cilantro

½ cup chopped onion

2 tsp cumin

8 oz diced green chilies

1 lb cooked ground turkey

Instructions:

Place the onion, chopped cilantro and diced green chilies into a pan and saute for around 3 minutes. Set this aside.

Cook the ground turkey through and then add the cumin, chili powder and salt,

Combine the ingredients that you set aside with the cooked ground turkey

Remove the tops of the peppers and remove all the seeds inside. Set them inside of a baking dish.

Split the turkey mixture between the peppers.

You should set your oven to 350°F.

Place the peppers into the oven for an hour, or until the turkey has cooked through. Enjoy!

Servings: 6

Nutrition:

- **Calories:** 337
- **Net Carbs:** 12 g
- **Proteins:** 24 g
- **Fats:** 14 g

Ketogenic Meal Plans for Intermittent fasting

Now that you have the recipes and know what the five different intermittent fasting cycles require, here are five ketogenic meal plans that will help you get started. There will be a week-long meal plan for each of the fasting cycles involving the recipes used from this book. They will each fit into a keto diet plan that consists of 1700 calories. This is an average figure, and you should figure out your own macro numbers.

Leangains

Monday

- Breakfast 12:00 pm – 1:00 pm
  - Chili Cheese Muffins
- Lunch 4:00 pm – 5:00 pm
  - Fish Sticks
- Dinner 8:00 pm – 9:00 pm
  - Shepherd's Pie

Fasting: Monday 9:00 pm – Tuesday 12:00 pm

Tuesday

- Breakfast 12:00 pm – 1:00 pm
  - Porridge
- Lunch 4:00 pm – 5:00 pm
  - Thai Chicken Wrap
- Dinner 8:00 pm – 9:00 pm

o   Beef Brisket

Fasting: Tuesday 9:00 pm – Wednesday 12:00 pm

Wednesday

- Breakfast 12:00 pm – 1:00 pm
  - o   Italian Omelet
- Lunch 4:00 pm – 5:00 pm
  - o   Meatballs
- Dinner 8:00 pm – 9:00 pm
  - o   Stuffed Peppers

Fasting: Wednesday 9:00 pm – Thursday 12:00 pm

Thursday

- Breakfast 12:00 pm – 1:00 pm
  - o   Sausage and Kale Hash
- Lunch 4:00 pm – 5:00 pm
  - o   Salmon Burger
- Dinner 8:00 pm – 9:00 pm
  - o   Stir Fry

Fasting: Thursday 9:00 pm – Friday 12:00 pm

Friday

- Breakfast 12:00 pm – 1:00 pm
  - o   Brie and Bacon Frittata
- Lunch 4:00 pm – 5:00 pm
  - o   Curried Shrimp
- Dinner 8:00 pm – 9:00 pm

- o Chicken and Cauliflower

Fasting: Friday 9:00 pm – Saturday 12:00 pm

Saturday

- Breakfast 12:00 pm – 1:00 pm
  - o Italian Omelet
- Lunch 4:00 pm – 5:00 pm
  - o Thai Chicken Wrap
- Dinner 8:00 pm – 9:00 pm
  - o Stir Fry

Fasting: Saturday 9:00 pm – Sunday 12:00 pm

Sunday

- Breakfast 12:00 pm – 1:00 pm
  - o Porridge
- Lunch 4:00 pm – 5:00 pm
  - o Salmon Burger
- Dinner 8:00 pm – 9:00 pm
  - o Stuffed Peppers

Fasting: Sunday 9:00 pm – Monday 12:00 pm

Eat Stop Eat

Monday

- Breakfast 7:00 am – 8:00 am
  - o Italian Omelet
- Lunch 12:00 pm – 1:00 pm

- o   Thai Chicken Wrap
- Dinner 6:00 pm – 7:00 pm
  - o   Stir Fry

Tuesday

- Breakfast 7:00 am – 8:00 am
  - o   Sausage and Kale Hash
- Lunch 12:00 pm – 1:00 pm
  - o   Salmon Burger
- Dinner 6:00 pm – 7:00 pm
  - o   Shepherd's Pie

Fasting: Tuesday 7:00 pm – Wednesday 7:00 pm

Wednesday

- Dinner 7:00 pm – 8:00 pm
  - o   Chicken and Cauliflower

Thursday

- Breakfast 7:00 am – 8:00 am
  - o   Porridge
- Lunch 12:00 pm – 1:00 pm
  - o   Thai Chicken Wrap
- Dinner 6:00 pm – 7:00 pm
  - o   Beef Brisket

Friday

- Breakfast 7:00 am – 8:00 am
  - o   Chili Cheese Muffins

- Lunch 12:00 pm – 1:00 pm
  - Fish Sticks
- Dinner 6:00 pm – 7:00 pm
  - Shepherd's Pie

Fasting: Friday 7:00 pm – Saturday 7:00 pm

Saturday

- Dinner 7:00 pm – 8:00 pm
  - Stuffed Peppers

Sunday

- Breakfast 7:00 am – 8:00 am
  - Italian Omelet
- Lunch 12:00 pm – 1:00 pm
  - Thai Chicken Wrap
- Dinner 6:00 pm – 7:00 pm
  - Stir Fry

5:2 Diet

Monday (fast day, 500-600 calories)

- Breakfast 8:00 am – 9:00 am
  - Jalapeno Popper Egg Cups
- Lunch 12:00pm – 1:00 pm
  - Kale Chips
- Dinner 6:00 pm – 7:00 pm
  - Fried Mac and Cheese

Tuesday

- Breakfast 8:00 am – 9:00 am
  - o Chili Cheese Muffins
- Lunch 12:00 pm – 1:00 pm
  - o Fish Sticks
- Dinner 6:00 pm – 7:00 pm
  - o Shepherd's Pie

Wednesday

- Breakfast 8:00 am – 9:00 am
  - o Brie and Bacon Frittata
- Lunch 12:00 pm – 1:00 pm
  - o Curried Shrimp
- Dinner 6:00 pm – 7:00 pm
  - o Chicken and Cauliflower

Thursday (fast day, 500-600 calories)

- Breakfast 8:00 am – 9:00 am
  - o Bacon and Cheese Cauliflower Muffins
- Lunch 12:00 pm – 1:00 pm
  - o Smoked Salmon and Goat Cheese Bites
- Dinner 6:00 pm – 7:00 pm
  - o Spiced Bacon Deviled Eggs

Friday

- Breakfast 8:00 am – 9:00 am
  - o Porridge

- Lunch 12:00 pm – 1:00 pm
  - Thai Chicken Wrap
- Dinner 6:00 pm – 7:00 pm
  - Beef Brisket

Saturday

- Breakfast 8:00 am – 9:00 am
  - Sausage and Kale Hash
- Lunch 12:00 pm – 1:00 pm
  - Salmon Burger
- Dinner 6:00 pm – 7:00 pm
  - Stir Fry

Sunday

- Breakfast 8:00 am – 9:00 am
  - Chili Cheese Muffins
- Lunch 12:00 pm – 1:00 pm
  - Fish Sticks
- Dinner 6:00 pm – 7:00 pm
  - Shepherd's Pie

Alternate Day Fasting

Sunday

- Breakfast 8:00 am – 9:00 am
  - Chili Cheese Muffins
- Lunch 12:00 pm – 1:00 pm

- o Fish Sticks:
- Dinner 6:00 pm – 7:00 pm
  - o Shepherd's Pie:

Monday (fast day, 400-500 calories)

- Breakfast 8:00 am – 9:00 am
  - o Bacon and Cheese Cauliflower Muffins
- Lunch 12:00 pm – 1:00 pm
  - o Kale Chips
- Dinner 6:00 pm – 7:00 pm
  - o Spiced Bacon Deviled Eggs

Tuesday

- Breakfast 8:00 am – 9:00 am
  - o Brie and Bacon Frittata
- Lunch 12:00 pm – 1:00 pm
  - o Curried Shrimp
- Dinner 6:00 pm – 7:00 pm
  - o Chicken and Cauliflower

Wednesday (fast day, 400-500 calories)

- Breakfast 8:00 am – 9:00 am
  - o Jalapeno Popper Egg Cups
- Lunch 12:00 pm – 1:00 pm
  - o Feta and Bacon Bites
- Dinner 6:00 pm – 7:00 pm
  - o Fried Mac and Cheese

Thursday

- Breakfast 8:00 am – 9:00 am
  - o Porridge
- Lunch 12:00 pm – 1:00 pm
  - o Thai Chicken Wrap
- Dinner 6:00 pm – 7:00 pm
  - o Beef Brisket

Friday (fast day, 400-500 calories)

- Breakfast 8:00 am – 9:00 am
  - o Goat Cheese Tomato Tarts
- Lunch 12:00 pm – 1:00 pm
  - o Smoked Salmon and Goat Cheese Bites
- Dinner 6:00 pm – 7:00 pm
  - o Pizza Chips

Saturday

- Breakfast 8:00 am – 9:00 am
  - o Porridge:
- Lunch 12:00 pm – 1:00 pm
  - o Thai Chicken Wrap
- Dinner 6:00 pm – 7:00 pm
  - o Beef Brisket

16:8 Diet

Monday:

- Breakfast 12:00 pm – 2:00 pm
  - Chili Cheese Muffins
- Lunch 4:00 pm – 5:00 pm
  - Fish Sticks
- Dinner 7:00 pm – 8:00 pm
  - Shepherd's Pie

Fasting: Monday 8:00 pm – Tuesday 12:00 pm

Tuesday:

- Breakfast 12:00 pm – 2:00 pm
  - Porridge
- Lunch 4:00 pm – 5:00 pm
  - Thai Chicken Wrap
- Dinner 7:00 pm – 8:00 pm
  - Beef Brisket

Fasting: Tuesday 8:00 pm – Wednesday 12:00 pm

Wednesday:

- Breakfast 12:00 pm – 2:00 pm
  - Italian Omelet
- Lunch 4:00 pm – 5:00 pm
  - Meatballs
- Dinner 7:00 pm – 8:00 pm
  - Stuffed Peppers

Fasting: Wednesday 8:00 pm – Thursday 12:00 pm

Thursday:

- Breakfast 12:00 pm – 2:00 pm
  - Sausage and Kale Hash
- Lunch 4:00 pm – 5:00 pm
  - Salmon Burger
- Dinner 7:00 pm – 8:00 pm
  - Stir Fry

Fasting: Thursday 8:00 pm – Friday 12:00 pm

Friday:

- Breakfast 12:00 pm – 2:00 pm
  - Brie and Bacon Frittata
- Lunch 4:00 pm – 5:00 pm
  - Curried Shrimp
- Dinner 7:00 pm – 8:00 pm
  - Chicken and Cauliflower

Fasting: Friday 8:00 pm – Saturday 12:00 pm

Saturday:

- Breakfast 12:00 pm – 2:00 pm
  - Italian Omelet
- Lunch 4:00 pm – 5:00 pm
  - Thai Chicken Wrap
- Dinner: 7:00 pm – 8:00 pm
  - Stir Fry

Fasting: Saturday 8:00 pm – Sunday 12:00 pm

Sunday:

- Breakfast 12:00 pm – 2:00 pm
    - Porridge
- Lunch 4:00 pm – 5:00 pm
    - Salmon Burger
- Dinner 7:00 pm – 8:00 pm
    - Stuffed Peppers

Fasting: Sunday 8:00 pm – Monday 12:00 pm

Conclusion

Congratulations and thank you for making it through to the end of, 'Intermittent Fasting + Keto Diet: Ketogenic Meal Plans For Intermittent Fasting, The Ultimate Fat Burning Combination'. I hope you found this book enjoyable and that it was able to provide you with all the tools you need to achieve your goals of adopting a new and healthy lifestyle.

You have just learned a lot of new information about the amazing benefits that come with intermittent fasting and the ketogenic diet. You've learned how you can combine these so you can implement them into your daily life, you have multiple structured schedules for intermittent fasting and meal plans, and heaps of ketogenic recipes at hand to help you achieve your goals. This may seem like a lot of information to absorb at the moment, but if you go through and follow these meal plans you won't fail. Once you figure out the best strategy for your needs, things will begin to fall into place.

Remember to let your body get used to the ketogenic diet for the first two weeks before starting the intermittent fasting cycles. When you first start the change, it may seem difficult, but trust me, it will become easier. You will be able to follow the rules and the diet without even thinking about it. It will become second nature to you, and it won't even feel like a diet anymore. Your friends and family will all start seeing the massive health changes you're going through and want to know exactly what you're doing.

Get started by deciding which intermittent fasting plan will work best for you, and then pick a day to begin your journey. Many people have reaped the benefits from the ancient science of intermittent fasting and the greatly revered ketogenic diet, in combination these two diet patterns work wonders for your health. So why not give it a try yourself?

Finally, if you enjoyed this book, it would be greatly appreciated if you could share your thoughts and leave an Amazon review for me!

Thank you and good luck!

Check Out My Other Books

Below you'll find two of my other books on intermittent fasting that are popular on Amazon and Kindle as well. Simply click on the links below to check them out. Alternatively, you can visit my author page on Amazon to see other work done by me.

- Intermittent Fasting For Women: Beat The Food Craving, And Get That Weight Shaving

- Intermittent Fasting: The Uncovered Celebrity Secret To Accelerate Weight Loss, Build Lean Muscle Fast, And Secure Your Healthiest Body And Mind

If the links do not work, for whatever reason, you can simply search for these titles on the Amazon website to find them.

94116753R00057

Made in the USA
Lexington, KY
23 July 2018